CONTENTS

EXPLORING THE INVISIBLE THREATS: MICROPLASTICS AND ZOMBIE CELLS

EXPLORING THE INVISIBLE THREATS
THREATS
Microplastics and Zombie Cells
ROBERT ANDERSON LOVE WINS

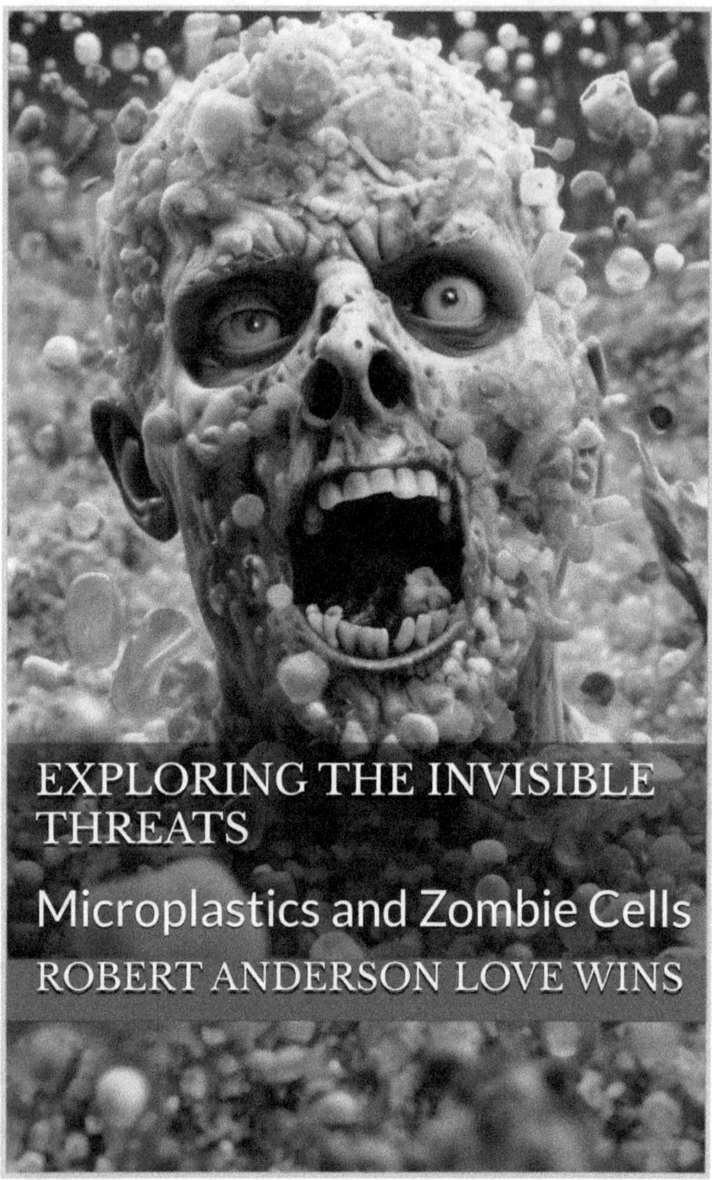

Index:

senescent cells for therapeutic purposes

5. Chapter 4: Linking Microplastics and Zombie Cells

- Potential connections between microplastics and senescence

- Shared mechanisms of toxicity and impact on human health

- Future research directions and implications for public health

6. Conclusion

- Summary of key findings

- Call to action for addressing the threats of microplastics and senescent cells

- Suggestions for further reading and resources

By organizing the content in this index, readers will have a clear roadmap of the topics covered in the book and how they are interconnected.

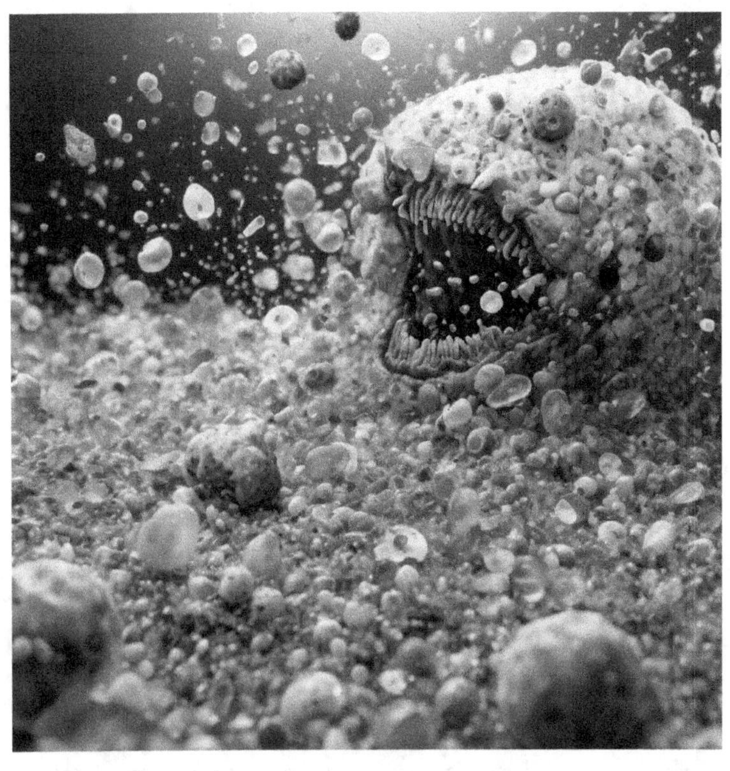

INTRODUCTION:

Invisible threats surround us every day, posing risks to our health and the environment. Two of these threats, microplastics and zombie cells, have gained increasing attention in recent years. Microplastics, tiny plastic particles that pervade our environment, and zombie cells, dysfunctional cells that accumulate in our bodies, both have the potential to impact human health in ways we are only beginning to understand.

This book delves into the world of microplastics and zombie cells, exploring their origins, impact, and the connections between these seemingly disparate phenomena. By shedding light on these invisible threats, we aim to raise awareness about their potential risks and inspire action to mitigate their effects. Through a combination of scientific research, expert insights, and real-world examples, we seek to provide a comprehensive understanding of these topics and their implications for human health.

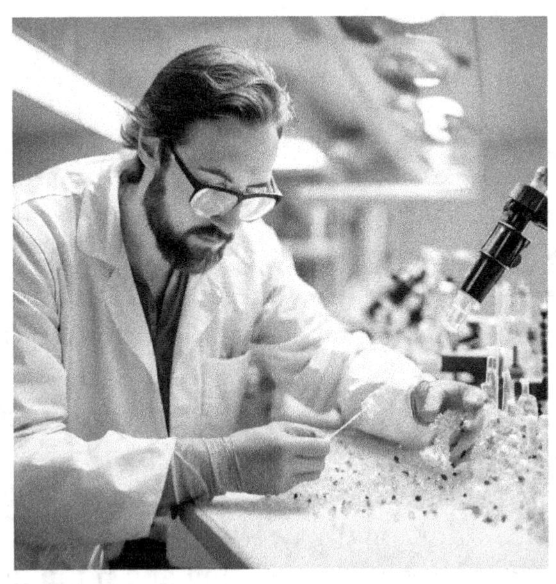

OVERVIEW:

Chapter 1 introduces the concept of microplastics, delving into their definition, sources, and the extensive reach of their pollution. We will examine the impact of microplastics on the environment, including their effects on marine life and ecosystems, as well as their potential to enter the food chain and ultimately impact human health. Furthermore, we will explore the various routes through which we are exposed to microplastics, from ingestion to inhalation, and the potential consequences of this exposure.

Chapter 2 focuses on the health effects of microplastics. Drawing from the latest research, we will delve into the potential risks associated with microplastic exposure, including inflammation, oxidative stress, and potential disruptions to the endocrine system. We will explore the ongoing scientific investigations into the impacts of microplastics on human health, highlighting the need for continued research and understanding in this field. Additionally, we will explore strategies to reduce microplastic pollution and minimize our exposure to these harmful particles.

In Chapter 3, our attention turns to zombie cells, also known as senescent cells. We will explore the biological mechanisms behind senescence and its role in the aging process. By examining the senescence-associated secretory phenotype (SASP), we will delve into the detrimental effects of zombie cells on our health, including their contribution to chronic inflammation and age-related diseases. We will also explore current research on senolytics, a promising field aiming to selectively eliminate senescent cells while preserving healthy cells, and its potential implications for extending healthspan and lifespan.

Chapter 4 bridges the gap between microplastics and zombie cells, exploring potential connections and shared mechanisms of toxicity. By examining the current understanding of how microplastics and senescent cells impact human health, we aim to shed light on the potential synergistic effects and the need for further research in this interdisciplinary field. We will discuss the implications of these connections for public health and emphasize the urgency of addressing both microplastics and zombie cells to safeguard our well-being.

In conclusion, this book aims to provide a comprehensive exploration of the invisible threats posed by microplastics and zombie cells. By unraveling the complexities of these phenomena and highlighting their potential impact on human health, we hope to inspire action and foster a deeper understanding of the risks we face. It is our belief that through knowledge and collective effort, we can mitigate these threats and pave the way for a healthier and more sustainable future.

CHAPTER 1: MICROPLASTICS

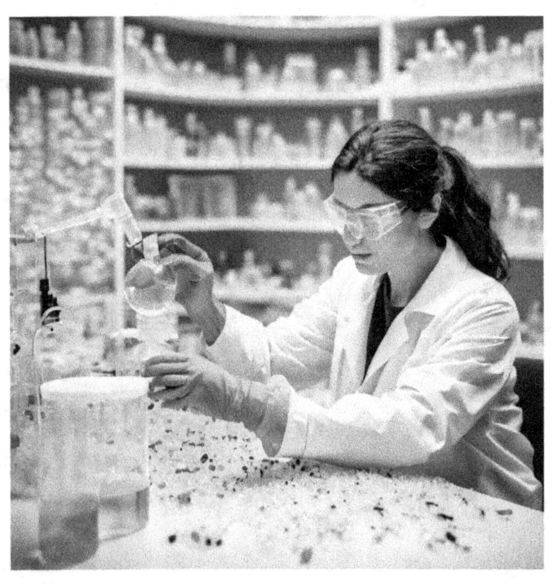

INTRODUCTION:

In today's modern world, plastic has become an integral part of our daily lives. From packaging materials to household items, plastic is everywhere. However, with the convenience of plastic comes a hidden threat: microplastics. In this chapter, we will explore the world of microplastics, understanding their definition, sources, and the extensive reach of their pollution. We will delve into the impact of microplastics on the environment, including their effects on marine life and ecosystems, as well as their potential to enter the food chain and ultimately impact human health. Furthermore, we will explore the various routes through which we are exposed to microplastics, from ingestion to inhalation, and the potential consequences of this exposure.

1.1 WHAT ARE MICROPLASTICS?

To understand the threat of microplastics, we must first grasp their definition. Microplastics are tiny plastic particles that are less than 5 millimeters in size. They can be either primary microplastics, which are intentionally manufactured at a small size, or secondary microplastics, which result from the breakdown of larger plastic items. These particles can take various forms, such as microbeads in personal care products, fibers from synthetic clothing, or fragments from plastic bags and bottles. Due to their small size, they are easily overlooked but pose significant risks to the environment and human health.

1.2 SOURCES OF MICROPLASTIC POLLUTION

Microplastics originate from a multitude of sources, with human activities being the primary contributors. One major source is the improper disposal of plastic waste. When plastic items, such as bottles or bags, break down in the environment, they fragment into smaller and smaller pieces, eventually becoming microplastics. Additionally, microbeads, which are tiny plastic particles used in personal care products like face scrubs and toothpaste, are another significant source of microplastic pollution. Synthetic textiles, such as polyester and nylon, shed microfibers during washing, which contribute to the release of microplastics into the environment. Other sources include industrial processes, such as plastic manufacturing, and the degradation of fishing gear and other plastic debris in the oceans.

1.3 IMPACT OF MICROPLASTICS ON THE ENVIRONMENT

Microplastics have a profound impact on the environment, particularly in aquatic ecosystems. When microplastics enter rivers, lakes, and oceans, they can be ingested by marine organisms, resulting in a cascade of ecological consequences. Marine animals, from plankton to fish and marine mammals, can mistake microplastics for food, leading to internal injuries, blockages, and even death. Microplastics can also accumulate in the tissues of these organisms, potentially entering the food chain and impacting larger predators, including humans.

Furthermore, microplastics pose a threat to delicate marine ecosystems, such as coral reefs and seagrass beds. They can smother and suffocate these habitats, disrupting the intricate balance of marine life. Additionally, microplastics can transport harmful chemicals, such as pesticides and persistent organic pollutants, acting as carriers and potentially contaminating organisms that ingest them.

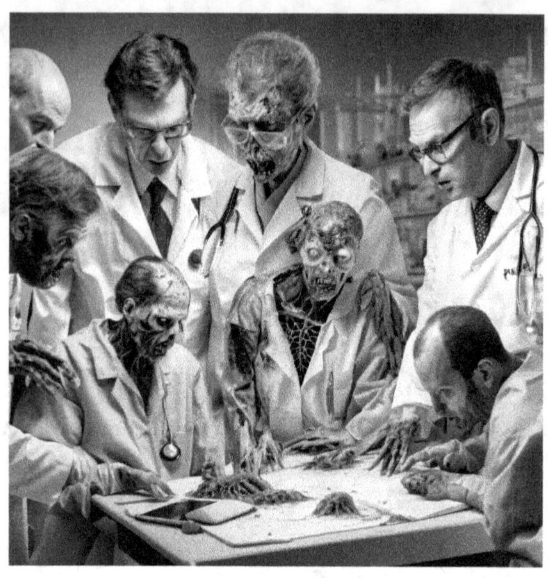

1.4 ROUTES OF EXPOSURE TO MICROPLASTICS

Humans are exposed to microplastics through various routes. One of the primary routes is through the consumption of contaminated food and water. Microplastics can be present in seafood, including fish, shellfish, and mollusks, as well as in drinking water and even bottled water. Inhalation is another potential route of exposure, as microplastics can become airborne and be inhaled, particularly in indoor environments where synthetic fibers are prevalent. Moreover, microplastics can be absorbed through the skin, primarily from personal care products containing microbeads or through direct contact with contaminated surfaces.

1.5 POTENTIAL CONSEQUENCES OF MICROPLASTIC EXPOSURE

While the full extent of the health impacts of microplastics on the human body is still being studied, several potential risks have emerged from scientific research. Microplastics can cause physical damage to organs and tissues, leading to inflammation and oxidative stress. In addition, the chemicals associated with microplastics, such as phthalates and bisphenol A, have been linked to endocrine disruption and potential long-term health effects.

Furthermore, microplastics may serve as vehicles for harmful bacteria and other pathogens, potentially contributing to the spread of infectious diseases. With the increasing prevalence of microplastics in the environment and their potential to accumulate in the human body, it is crucial to understand the potential risks they pose to human health.

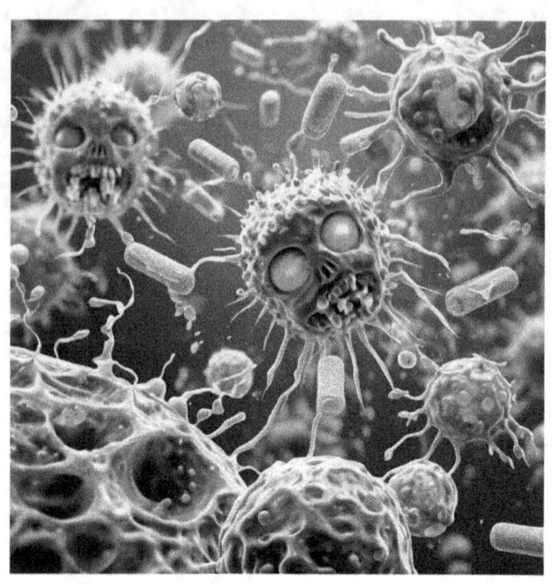

CONCLUSION:

In this chapter, we have explored the world of microplastics, understanding their definition, sources, and the extensive reach of their pollution. We have delved into the impact of microplastics on the environment, including their effects on marine life and ecosystems, as well as their potential to enter the food chain and ultimately impact human health. Furthermore, we have discussed the various routes through which we are exposed to microplastics and the potential consequences of this exposure. As we move forward in this book, it is essential to recognize the urgent need to address microplastic pollution and minimize our exposure to protect both the environment and our own well-being.

CHAPTER 2: HEALTH EFFECTS OF MICROPLASTICS

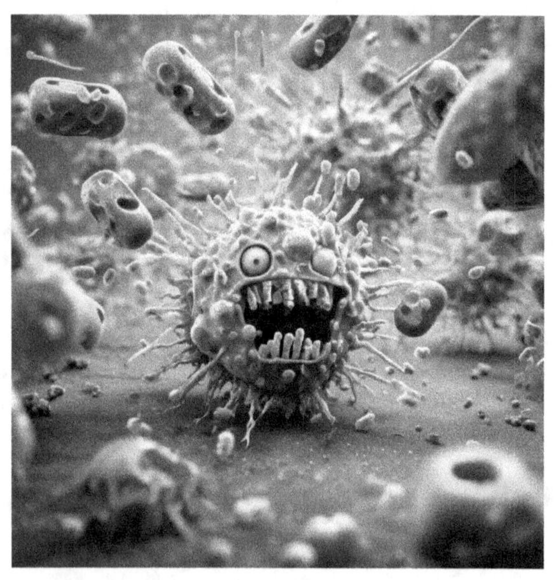

INTRODUCTION:

In Chapter 1, we explored the world of microplastics, understanding their sources and the extensive pollution they cause. Now, in Chapter 2, we will focus on the potential health effects of microplastics. While our understanding is still evolving, scientific research has shed light on the potential risks associated with microplastic exposure. We will delve into these risks, exploring the impact of microplastics on human health. By examining the latest research and understanding the mechanisms through which microplastics can affect our bodies, we aim to raise awareness about the potential consequences of this invisible threat.

2.1 POTENTIAL HEALTH RISKS ASSOCIATED WITH MICROPLASTIC EXPOSURE

Microplastics have the potential to impact human health in various ways. While more research is needed to fully understand the extent of these risks, several potential health effects have emerged from scientific studies. One of the primary concerns is inflammation, as microplastics can trigger an immune response in the body. Chronic inflammation has been linked to a range of health issues, including cardiovascular disease, diabetes, and neurodegenerative disorders.

Another potential risk is oxidative stress, which

occurs when there is an imbalance between the production of harmful reactive oxygen species (ROS) and the body's ability to detoxify them. Microplastics can generate ROS, leading to oxidative damage to cells and tissues. This oxidative stress can contribute to various diseases, including cancer, aging-related conditions, and neurodegenerative disorders.

Furthermore, microplastics contain or can absorb chemicals from the environment, such as phthalates, bisphenol A, and polycyclic aromatic hydrocarbons (PAHs). These chemicals have been associated with endocrine disruption, potentially affecting hormone regulation and reproductive health. Additionally, studies have suggested that microplastics may disrupt the gut microbiome, the collection of microorganisms that play a crucial role in digestion, immune function, and overall health.

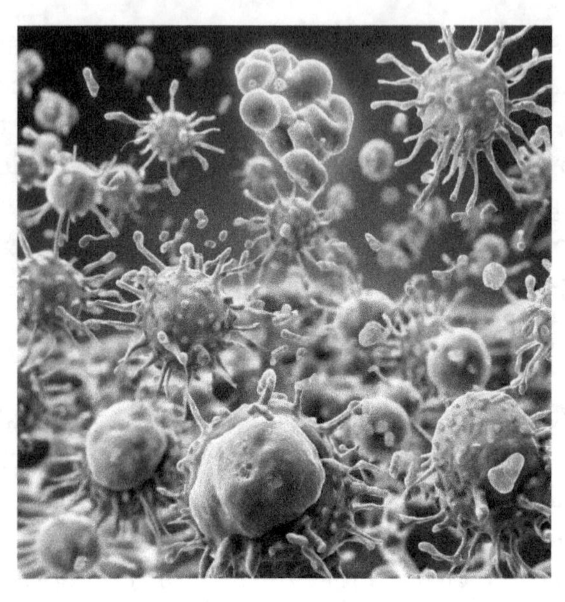

2.2 RESEARCH ON THE IMPACT OF

MICROPLASTICS ON HUMAN HEALTH

In recent years, scientists have been actively researching the potential health effects of microplastics. Studies have been conducted to understand the presence of microplastics in various tissues and organs, such as the gut, lung, liver, kidney, and even the placenta. These studies have provided evidence of microplastic accumulation in these tissues, raising concerns about the potential long-term consequences.

Animal studies have also provided valuable insights into the health effects of microplastics. Research conducted on various animal species, including fish, birds, and mammals, has shown adverse effects on reproduction, development, and immune function. These findings underscore the potential risks that microplastics pose to ecosystems and human health.

Human epidemiological studies are another crucial aspect of research in this field. These studies aim to understand the relationship between microplastic exposure and health outcomes in human populations. While the field is relatively new, preliminary studies have shown associations between microplastic exposure and biomarkers of inflammation, oxidative stress, and endocrine disruption. However, further research is needed to establish causal relationships and determine the specific health impacts of microplastics on humans.

2.3 STRATEGIES TO REDUCE MICROPLASTIC POLLUTION AND EXPOSURE

Given the potential risks associated with microplastics, it is crucial to take action to reduce both microplastic pollution and our exposure to these particles. Several strategies can be implemented at various levels:

1. Individual actions: By adopting sustainable lifestyle choices, we can reduce our contribution to microplastic pollution. This includes minimizing the use of single-use plastics, choosing natural fibers over synthetic ones, properly disposing of plastic waste, and supporting initiatives that promote plastic-free alternatives.

2. Industry and policy changes: Governments and industries play a critical role in addressing microplastic pollution. Implementing regulations to ban or restrict the use of microbeads in personal care products, promoting the development of eco-friendly packaging materials, and investing in recycling technologies are some measures that can be taken.

3. Research and innovation: Continued research is essential to deepen our understanding of microplastics and their impacts. This includes developing improved detection and monitoring methods, studying the fate and transport of microplastics in the environment, and exploring innovative solutions for microplastic removal.

CONCLUSION:

In this chapter, we explored the potential health effects of microplastics, shedding light on the risks associated with exposure to these particles. While our understanding is still evolving, scientific research has highlighted the potential for inflammation, oxidative stress, endocrine disruption, and gut microbiome disruption. Animal studies and human epidemiological studies have provided valuable insights into the impacts of microplastics on health. To mitigate these risks, it is crucial to implement strategies at individual, industry, and policy levels to reduce microplastic pollution and minimize exposure. By taking action and supporting ongoing research, we can work towards safeguarding human health and the environment from the invisible threat of microplastics.

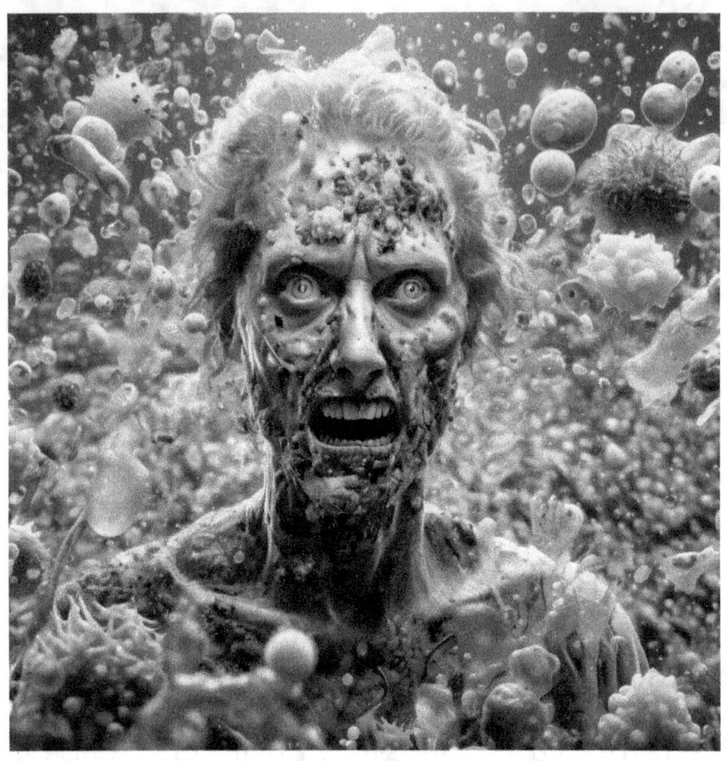

CHAPTER 3: ZOMBIE CELLS (SENESCENT CELLS)

INTRODUCTION:

In Chapter 2, we explored the potential health effects of microplastics, understanding the risks associated with exposure to these tiny particles. Now, in Chapter 3, we will delve into the world of zombie cells, also known as senescent cells. While microplastics pose a threat from external exposure, senescent cells are dysfunctional cells that accumulate within our bodies as we age. These cells can contribute to various age-related diseases and conditions, impacting our overall health and well-being. By understanding the biology of senescent cells and their role in the aging process, we can gain insights into potential strategies to improve health and extend lifespan.

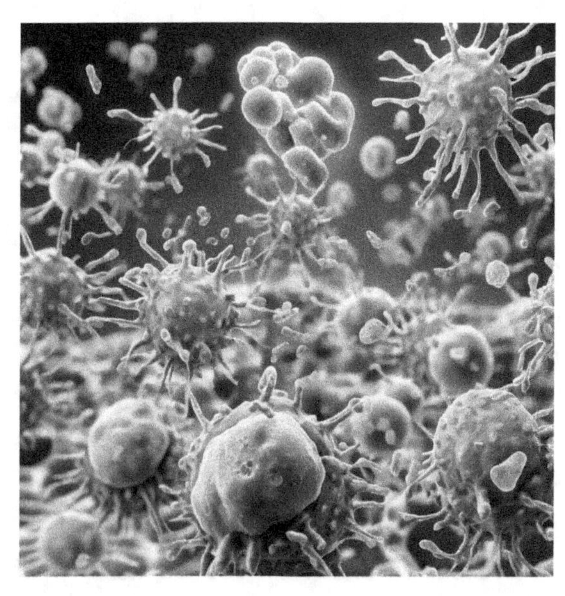

3.1 EXPLANATION OF SENESCENT

CELLS AND THEIR ROLE IN AGING

Senescent cells, often referred to as zombie cells, are cells that have irreversibly stopped dividing and are no longer functioning correctly. This cellular state is known as senescence, and it is a natural part of the aging process. Senescence can occur as a response to various stress factors, such as DNA damage, oxidative stress, or telomere shortening.

While senescence initially serves as a protective mechanism to prevent damaged cells from becoming cancerous, the accumulation of senescent cells can have detrimental effects on our health. Senescent cells can release inflammatory molecules and other harmful substances, disrupting the normal functioning of surrounding tissues and organs.

3.2 SENESCENCE-ASSOCIATED SECRETORY PHENOTYPE (SASP) AND ITS IMPACT ON HEALTH

One of the key features of senescent cells is their ability to secrete a range of molecules, collectively known as the senescence-associated secretory phenotype (SASP). The SASP includes various pro-inflammatory cytokines, growth factors, and matrix remodeling enzymes. While the SASP can be beneficial in the short term, promoting tissue repair and immune responses, its chronic activation can lead to chronic inflammation and tissue dysfunction.

Chronic inflammation associated with the SASP has been linked to the development of age-related diseases and conditions. It can contribute to the progression of cardiovascular disease, neurodegenerative disorders, metabolic disorders like diabetes, and even cancer. Additionally, the SASP can impair the function and regenerative capacity of neighboring healthy cells, further exacerbating tissue dysfunction.

3.3 CURRENT RESEARCH ON SENOLYTICS AND TARGETING SENESCENT CELLS FOR THERAPEUTIC PURPOSES

Given the detrimental effects of senescent cells on health, researchers have been actively exploring strategies to target and remove these cells from the body. This emerging field, known as senolytics, aims to develop therapies that selectively eliminate senescent cells while preserving healthy cells.

Senolytic compounds are molecules that can specifically induce apoptosis, or programmed cell death, in senescent cells. Various senolytics have been identified and tested in preclinical studies, demonstrating their potential to improve age-related health conditions. These compounds can target specific mechanisms involved in the survival and maintenance of senescent cells, ultimately leading to their elimination. Furthermore, other approaches such as immunotherapies and genetic interventions are being explored to target senescent cells.

While the field of senolytics is still in its early stages, initial studies in animal models have shown promising results. The selective removal of senescent cells has been associated with improved healthspan, reduced age-related disease burden, and even extended lifespan. However, further research is needed to optimize the efficacy and safety of these interventions before their application in humans.

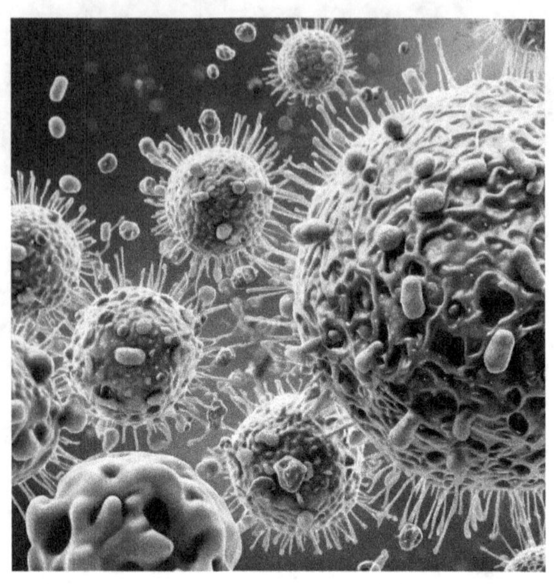

CONCLUSION:

In this chapter, we explored the world of senescent cells, understanding their biology and their role in the aging process. Senescent cells, also known as zombie cells, can accumulate in our bodies as a result of various stress factors and contribute to age-related diseases and tissue dysfunction. The senescence-associated secretory phenotype (SASP), characterized by the release of inflammatory molecules, plays a significant role in mediating the harmful effects of senescent cells.

Researchers are actively investigating strategies to target and eliminate senescent cells from the body, with the goal of improving health and extending lifespan. The field of senolytics shows promise, with the development of compounds that selectively induce apoptosis in senescent cells. Initial studies in animal models have demonstrated the potential benefits of senolytic interventions, including improved healthspan and reduced age-related disease burden. However, further research is necessary to refine these interventions and assess their safety and efficacy in humans.

By understanding the biology of senescent cells and the potential of targeting them, we can pave the way for novel therapeutic approaches to combat age-related diseases and promote healthy aging. The exploration of senescent cells offers hope for the future, as we strive to enhance the quality of life and extend the years of vitality.

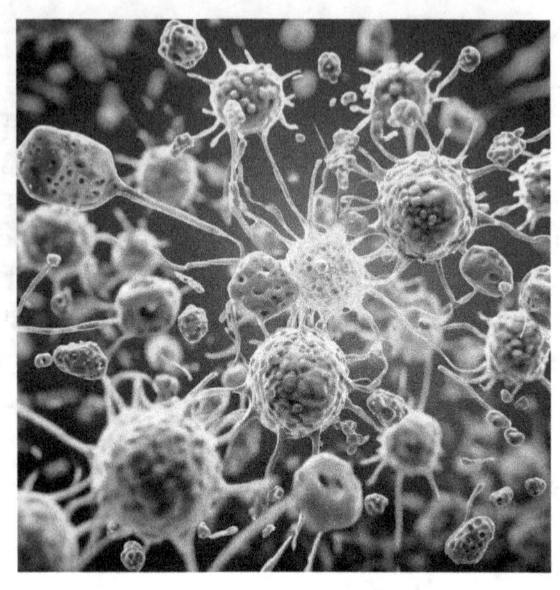

CHAPTER

4: LINKING MICROPLASTICS AND ZOMBIE CELLS

INTRODUCTION:

In the previous chapters, we explored the individual threats of microplastics and zombie cells, understanding their potential impact on human health. Now, in Chapter 4, we will bridge the gap between these seemingly disparate phenomena and explore the potential connections and shared mechanisms of toxicity. By examining the current understanding of how microplastics and senescent cells impact human health, we aim to shed light on the potential synergistic effects and the need for further research in this interdisciplinary field. We will discuss the implications of these connections for public health and emphasize the urgency of addressing both microplastics and zombie cells to safeguard our well-being.

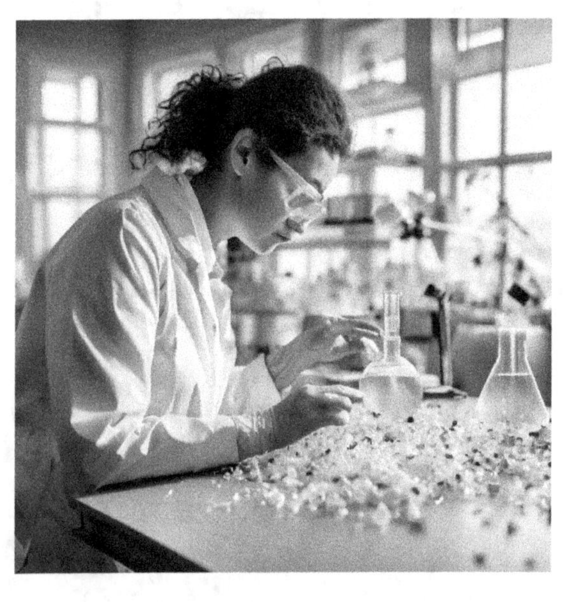

4.1 POTENTIAL

CONNECTIONS BETWEEN MICROPLASTICS AND SENESCENCE

While microplastics and senescent cells may appear to be unrelated, emerging research suggests potential connections between these two phenomena. One possible link is through the toxic chemicals associated with microplastics. Microplastics can absorb and transport harmful chemicals, including those known to induce senescence, such as oxidative stress-inducing compounds and endocrine disruptors. These chemicals can contribute to the accumulation of senescent cells in various tissues, potentially exacerbating age-related diseases and conditions.

Furthermore, chronic inflammation induced by microplastics and the senescence-associated secretory phenotype (SASP) can create a vicious cycle. Microplastics can trigger inflammation in the body, promoting the accumulation of senescent cells. In turn, senescent cells can release inflammatory molecules that perpetuate chronic inflammation, creating an environment conducive to the development and progression of age-related diseases.

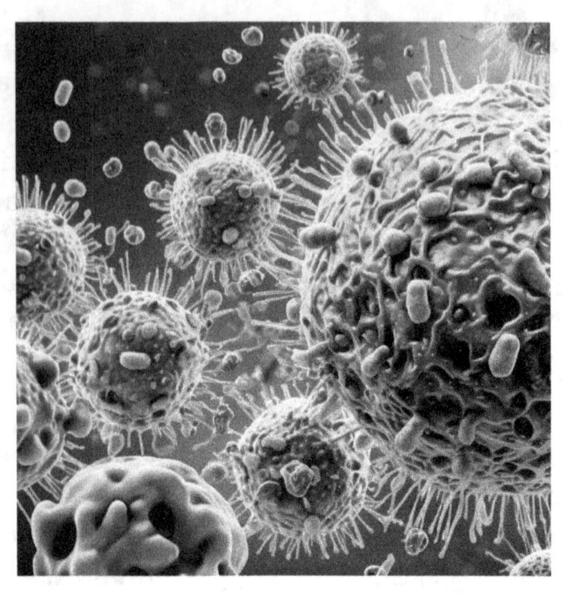

4.2 SHARED MECHANISMS OF TOXICITY

Microplastics and senescent cells share common mechanisms of toxicity that contribute to their impact on human health. One of these mechanisms is oxidative stress. Microplastics generate reactive oxygen species (ROS), leading to oxidative damage in cells and tissues. Senescent cells, too, contribute to oxidative stress through the SASP, which includes inflammatory molecules that can generate ROS. The cumulative oxidative stress caused by microplastics and senescent cells can lead to DNA damage, cellular dysfunction, and the progression of age-related diseases.

Another shared mechanism is inflammation. Microplastics can trigger an immune response in the body, leading to chronic inflammation. Senescent cells, through the SASP, release pro-inflammatory cytokines and chemokines, contributing to chronic inflammation as well. The chronic inflammation induced by both microplastics and senescent cells can disrupt normal tissue function and contribute to the development of various diseases.

4.3 FUTURE RESEARCH DIRECTIONS AND IMPLICATIONS FOR PUBLIC HEALTH

The potential connections between microplastics and senescent cells highlight the need for further research in this interdisciplinary field. Future studies should aim to investigate the specific mechanisms through which microplastics contribute to senescence and the impact of senescent cells on the accumulation and persistence of microplastics in the body. Understanding these connections can provide valuable insights into the complex interplay between environmental factors and cellular processes in the development of age-related diseases.

From a public health perspective, addressing both microplastics and senescent cells is essential for safeguarding human well-being. Efforts to reduce microplastic pollution and exposure should be coupled with strategies to target and eliminate senescent cells. By minimizing the accumulation of senescent cells and reducing chronic inflammation, we may be able to mitigate the impact of microplastics on cellular health and overall well-being.

Furthermore, interdisciplinary collaborations between environmental scientists, biologists, and medical researchers are crucial to comprehensively understand the connections between microplastics and senescent cells. By sharing knowledge, expertise, and resources, we can accelerate progress in this field and develop innovative solutions to address these invisible threats.

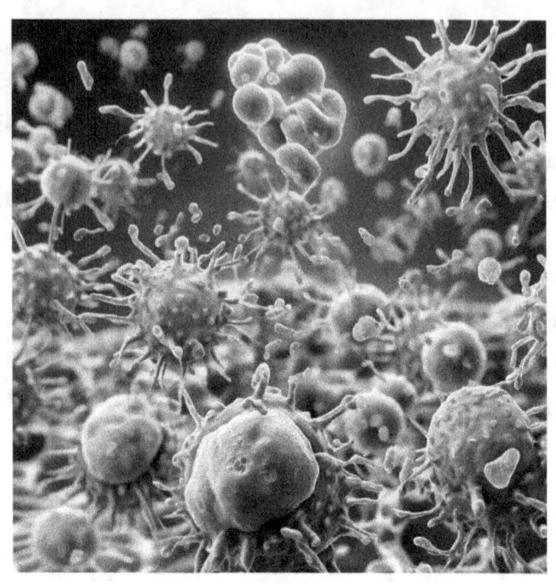

CONCLUSION:

In this chapter, we explored the potential connections and shared mechanisms of toxicity between microplastics and senescent cells. While seemingly unrelated, these phenomena have the potential to interact and contribute to the development and progression of age-related diseases. The toxic chemicals associated with microplastics can induce senescence, while senescent cells can promote the accumulation and persistence of microplastics in the body. Shared mechanisms of toxicity, such as oxidative stress and chronic inflammation, further contribute to their impact on human health.

Understanding these connections is crucial for developing comprehensive strategies to address both microplastics and senescent cells. By reducing microplastic pollution and exposure and targeting senescent cells, we can work towards mitigating the risks associated with these invisible threats. Further research and interdisciplinary collaborations are necessary to deepen our understanding and develop effective interventions. By addressing both microplastics and zombie cells, we can pave the way for a healthier future and improved quality of life.

CHAPTER 5: IMPLICATIONS FOR HUMAN HEALTH AND ENVIRONMENTAL WELL-BEING

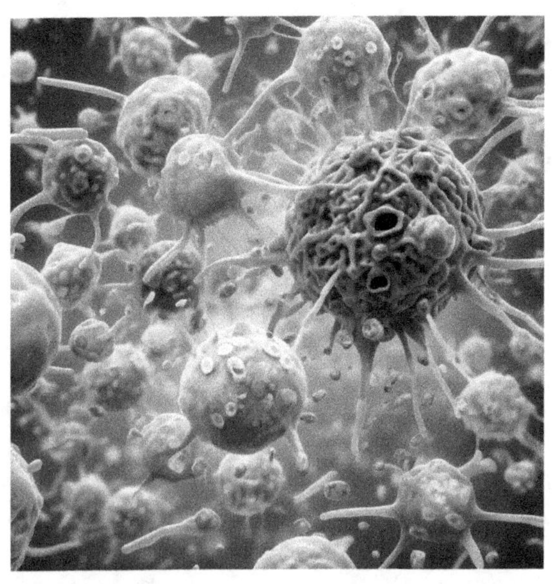

INTRODUCTION:

In the previous chapters, we explored the threats posed by microplastics and senescent cells individually, as well as the potential connections between these two phenomena. Now, in Chapter 5, we will delve into the broader implications of microplastics and zombie cells for human health and environmental well-being. By examining the cumulative impact of these invisible threats, we can gain a deeper understanding of the urgency to address these issues and the potential consequences of inaction. This chapter will explore the ripple effects of microplastics and senescent cells on ecosystems, public health, and the need for collective action to mitigate these challenges.

5.1 ECOLOGICAL AND ENVIRONMENTAL IMPLICATIONS

Microplastics have become pervasive pollutants in aquatic ecosystems, with far-reaching consequences for the environment. These tiny particles can accumulate in marine life, from small organisms like plankton to larger species like fish and marine mammals. The ingestion of microplastics can lead to physical harm, internal injuries, and even death. Additionally, microplastics can disrupt marine ecosystems, smothering delicate habitats like coral reefs and seagrass beds, and affecting the overall balance of marine life. The transport of harmful chemicals by microplastics further amplifies their ecological impact, potentially contaminating organisms and disrupting food chains.

Senescent cells, on the other hand, contribute to tissue dysfunction and impaired regeneration, which can have implications for ecological systems. In humans, the accumulation of senescent cells has been linked to age-related diseases, such as cardiovascular disease and neurodegenerative disorders. In animals, the presence of senescent cells can affect reproduction, development, and immune function, potentially impacting population dynamics and ecological interactions. Understanding the ecological implications of senescent cells can provide insights into the broader consequences of aging and the need to promote healthy aging in natural systems.

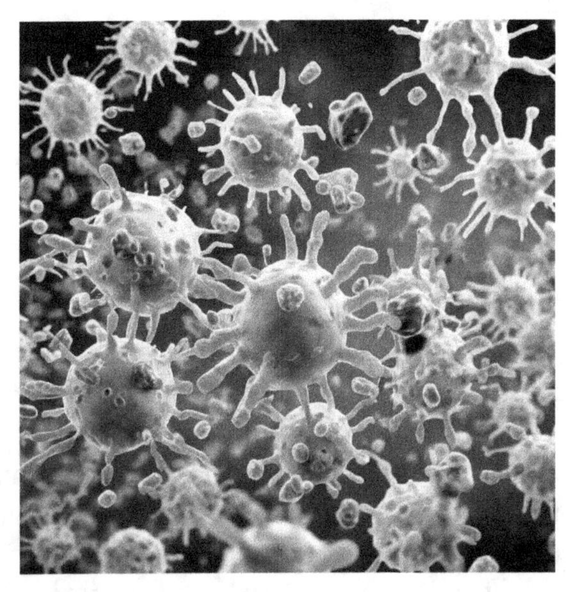

5.2 PUBLIC HEALTH

IMPLICATIONS

The threats posed by microplastics and senescent cells extend beyond the environment and have direct implications for human health. Microplastic pollution can impact human health through various routes of exposure, including ingestion, inhalation, and skin contact. The potential health risks associated with microplastics, such as inflammation, oxidative stress, and endocrine disruption, can contribute to the development and progression of chronic diseases, including cardiovascular disease, cancer, and neurodegenerative disorders. The increasing prevalence of microplastics in the environment and their potential to accumulate in the human body emphasize the need to address this issue to safeguard public health.

Similarly, senescent cells have significant implications for human health. The accumulation of senescent cells with age is associated with chronic inflammation, tissue dysfunction, and age-related diseases. Chronic inflammation induced by senescent cells can contribute to the progression of cardiovascular disease, neurodegenerative disorders, and other age-related conditions. By targeting senescent cells and reducing chronic inflammation, there is the potential to delay the onset of age-related diseases, improve healthspan, and enhance overall well-being.

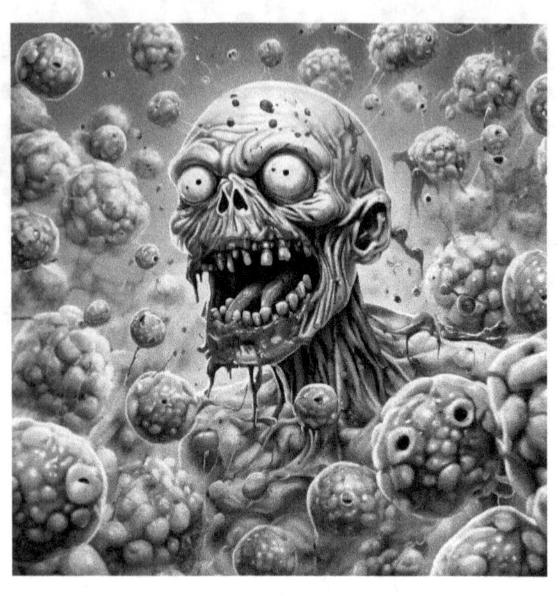

5.3 THE NEED FOR COLLECTIVE ACTION

The threats of microplastics and senescent cells require collective action at various levels to effectively address the challenges they pose. Individual actions, such as reducing plastic consumption, properly disposing of plastic waste, and adopting sustainable lifestyle choices, can contribute to reducing microplastic pollution. Supporting policies and regulations that promote alternatives to single-use plastics and encourage responsible waste management is also crucial.

Furthermore, collaboration between industries, governments, and researchers is essential to develop innovative solutions and technologies. Investing in research on microplastics and senescent cells can deepen our understanding of their impacts and inform the development of effective strategies. This interdisciplinary collaboration can lead to the development of environmentally friendly materials, improved waste management practices, and novel therapeutic approaches for targeting senescent cells.

Education and awareness initiatives are vital in empowering individuals and communities to take action. By raising awareness about the risks of microplastics and the importance of healthy aging, we can foster a collective sense of responsibility and drive change. Engaging with communities, schools, and businesses to promote sustainable practices and health-conscious behaviors can create a ripple effect of positive change.

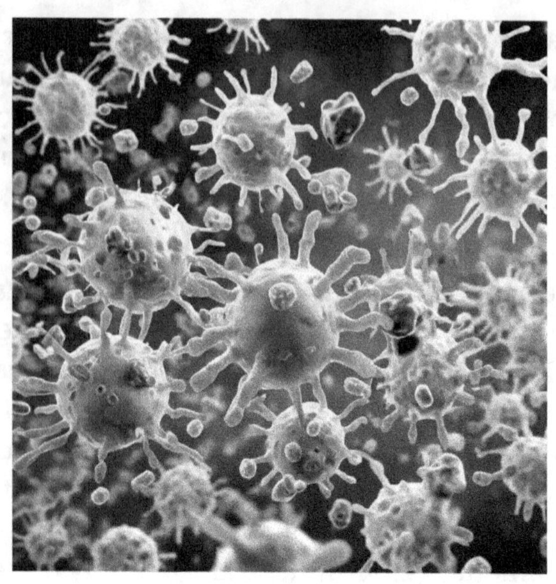

CONCLUSION:

In this chapter, we explored the broader implications of microplastics and senescent cells for human health and environmental well-being. The ecological impact of microplastics extends beyond marine life, affecting delicate habitats and disrupting ecosystems. Senescent cells, on the other hand, have implications for tissue dysfunction and age-related diseases in both humans and animals. Understanding these implications emphasizes the need for collective action to address these invisible threats.

Microplastics and senescent cells have direct implications for human health, contributing to chronic diseases and impairing overall well-being. The risks associated with microplastics and the accumulation of senescent cells underscore the urgency to address these issues. By taking collective action at individual, industry, and policy levels, we can mitigate the environmental and health impacts of microplastics and promote healthy aging.

Education, research, and collaboration are key to driving change. By raising awareness, investing in research, and fostering interdisciplinary collaborations, we can develop innovative solutions, promote sustainable practices, and improve public health outcomes. The challenges posed by microplastics and senescent cells require a comprehensive and concerted effort to protect our environment, enhance human health, and ensure a sustainable future for generations to come.

The invisible threats of microplastics and senescent cells have far-reaching implications for both human health and environmental well-being. Throughout this book, we have explored the individual dangers of these phenomena and the potential connections between them. Microplastics, with their pervasive presence in our environment, have the potential to enter our bodies through various routes and pose risks such as inflammation, oxidative stress, and endocrine disruption. Senescent cells, accumulating as we age, contribute to chronic inflammation and tissue dysfunction, leading to age-related diseases and impaired health.

The potential connections between microplastics and senescent cells highlight the complex interplay between our environment and cellular processes. It is becoming increasingly clear that the toxic chemicals associated with microplastics can induce senescence, while senescent cells can promote the accumulation and persistence of microplastics in the body. Shared mechanisms of toxicity, such as oxidative stress and chronic inflammation, further amplify their impact on human health.

The implications of microplastics and senescent cells extend beyond individual health. Microplastics have profound ecological consequences, affecting marine life and disrupting delicate ecosystems. Senescent cells can impact population dynamics and ecological interactions, potentially influencing the health of natural systems. The need to address these invisible threats is urgent, as they have significant implications for both our own well-being and the health of the planet.

Collective action is necessary to tackle the

challenges posed by microplastics and senescent cells. Individuals can make a difference by reducing plastic consumption, supporting sustainable practices, and promoting responsible waste management. Industries and governments play a crucial role in implementing regulations, investing in research, and developing innovative solutions. Collaboration between scientists, environmental experts, and health professionals is essential to deepen our understanding, drive innovation, and develop effective strategies.

Education and awareness are key to empowering individuals and communities to take action. By raising awareness about the risks of microplastics and the importance of healthy aging, we can foster a collective sense of responsibility and inspire positive change. Through education initiatives, community engagement, and sustainable practices, we can pave the way for a healthier future for both humans and the environment.

In conclusion, addressing the threats of microplastics and senescent cells requires a comprehensive and collaborative effort. By taking action at individual, industry, and policy levels, we can mitigate the risks, protect our environment, promote healthy aging, and ensure a sustainable future for generations to come. It is through our collective commitment and action that we can overcome these invisible threats and create a world where both human health and the environment thrive.

In this book, we have explored the invisible threats posed by microplastics and senescent cells, shedding light on their potential impact on human health and environmental well-being. We have uncovered the individual risks associated with microplastics and zombie cells, as well as the potential connections and shared mechanisms of toxicity between these two phenomena. Now, it's time to summarize our key findings and call to action for addressing these threats.

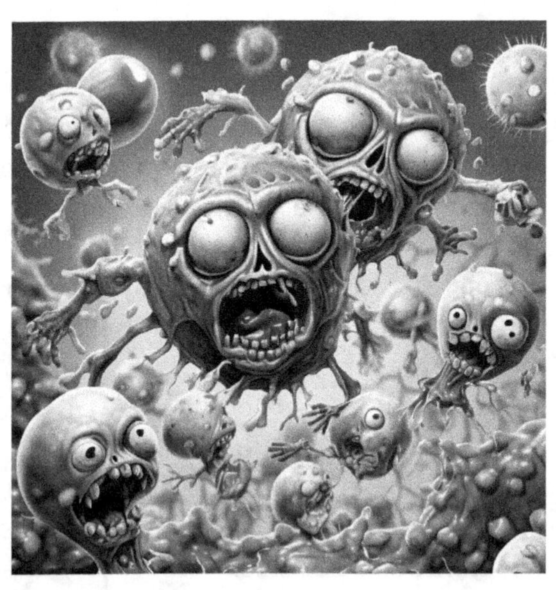

SUMMARY OF KEY FINDINGS:

Throughout this book, we have learned that microplastics are tiny plastic particles that can enter our bodies through various routes and have the potential to cause inflammation, oxidative stress, and endocrine disruption. These particles have pervasive pollution in the environment, impacting marine life and ecosystems. On the other hand, senescent cells, also known as zombie cells, accumulate in our bodies as we age and contribute to chronic inflammation and tissue dysfunction. Senescent cells have been linked to age-related diseases such as cardiovascular disease and neurodegenerative disorders.

We have explored the potential connections between microplastics and senescent cells, highlighting the role of toxic chemicals and shared mechanisms of toxicity, such as oxidative stress and chronic inflammation. Understanding these connections provides insights into the complex interplay between our environment and cellular processes and emphasizes the need for collective action.

CALL TO ACTION FOR ADDRESSING THE THREATS OF MICROPLASTICS AND SENESCENT CELLS:

The threats posed by microplastics and senescent cells require immediate action at various levels to protect human health and the environment. We must recognize the urgency of addressing these invisible threats and take responsibility for our role in mitigating their impact. Here are some key actions we can take:

1. Reduce plastic consumption: Minimize the use of single-use plastics and opt for sustainable alternatives. By reducing plastic consumption, we

can help decrease the amount of plastic waste that ends up in the environment.

2. Support policies and regulations: Advocate for policies that promote responsible waste management, ban or restrict the use of microbeads in personal care products, and encourage the development of eco-friendly materials and packaging.

3. Invest in research and innovation: Support research efforts aimed at understanding the impacts of microplastics and senescent cells on human health and the environment. By investing in research and innovation, we can develop effective strategies and technologies to address these challenges.

4. Promote education and awareness: Raise awareness about the risks of microplastics and the importance of healthy aging. Educate communities, schools, and businesses about sustainable practices, responsible waste management, and the potential consequences of these invisible threats.

5. Foster interdisciplinary collaborations: Encourage collaboration between scientists, environmental experts, health professionals, policymakers, and industry stakeholders. By

working together, we can leverage diverse expertise and resources to develop comprehensive solutions.

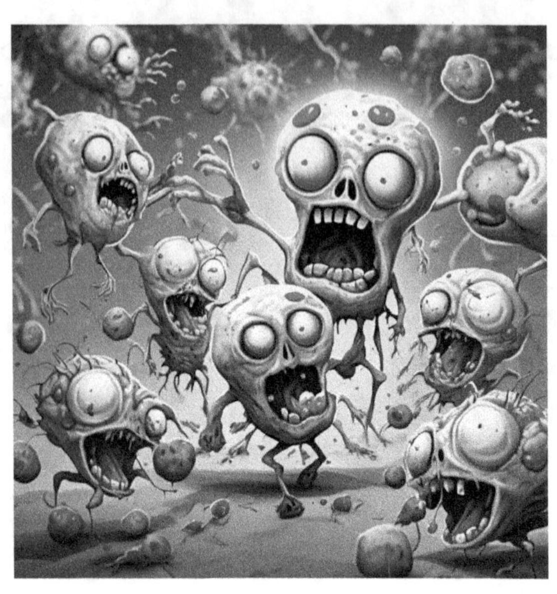

SUGGESTIONS FOR FURTHER RESOURCES:

To continue exploring the topics of microplastics and senescent cells, here are some suggestions for further reading and resources:

Websites such as environmental organizations,

and research institutions often provide valuable information and resources on microplastics, senescent cells, and related topics.

By staying informed and engaged, we can contribute to the collective effort to address the threats of microplastics and senescent cells, protect human health, and preserve the health of our planet for future generations.

Together, let us take action to reduce plastic pollution, promote healthy aging, and create a sustainable future for all.

The information contained in this book is Information is based on publicly available data. This book should be understood that while it strives to provide accurate and up-to-date information, this may not always reflect the most current research or medical guidelines. Therefore, it's always a good idea to consult a medical professional or trusted source for specific medical advice or information.

THIS BOOK ON MICROPLASTICS AND SENESCENT CELLS CAN BE A VALUABLE GIFT FOR A FRIEND FOR SEVERAL REASONS:

1. Awareness: This book provides a comprehensive understanding of the threats posed by microplastics and senescent cells, raising awareness about these invisible but significant challenges. By gifting this book, you can help your friend become more informed about these topics and their potential

impact on human health and the environment.

2. Education: The book offers a wealth of information and scientific research on microplastics and senescent cells, providing your friend with a deeper understanding of these phenomena. It explores the biology, sources, and potential health effects of microplastics, as well as the role of senescent cells in aging and age-related diseases. This knowledge can empower your friend to make informed choices and take action in their own lives.

3. Interdisciplinary perspective: The book bridges the gap between environmental science and human health, highlighting the interconnectedness of these fields. It explores the potential connections between microplastics and senescent cells, shedding light on shared mechanisms of toxicity and potential synergistic effects. By presenting an interdisciplinary perspective, the book encourages readers to consider the broader implications of these threats.

4. Call to action: The book not only informs but also calls for collective action to address the challenges of microplastics and senescent cells. It emphasizes the need for individual and collective efforts to reduce plastic pollution, promote sustainable practices, and invest in research and innovation. By gifting this book, you can inspire your friend to take

action and make a positive impact on their own health and the environment.

5. Thoughtful and meaningful gift: Giving a book that addresses important topics like microplastics and senescent cells shows that you care about your friend's well-being and the well-being of the planet. It demonstrates thoughtfulness and a desire to share valuable knowledge and insights. This book can spark meaningful conversations and discussions, fostering a deeper connection between you and your friend.

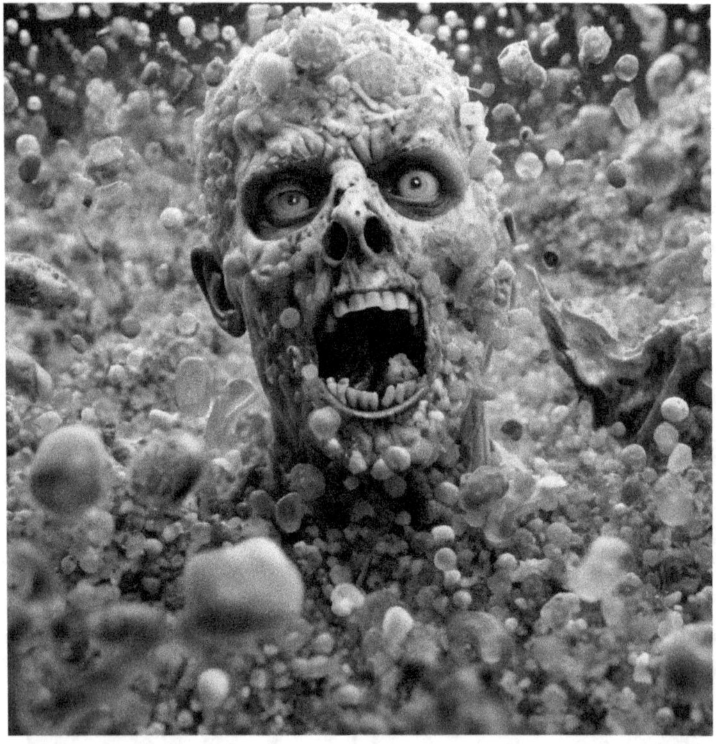

This book was given to you by

\-
\-\-

Phone# ___________________________

Overall, gifting this book on microplastics and senescent cells can be a meaningful gesture that promotes awareness, education, and action. It can empower your friend to make informed choices, take steps to reduce their environmental impact, and contribute to a healthier future for themselves and the planet.